The Magic of Makarasana
The Yoga posture that will

Transform your Life

Teresa Keast

Published by Teresa Keast
Copyright ©2025 Teresa Keast
All rights reserved

This book is licensed for your personal enjoyment only. It may not be re-sold. If you would like to share this book with another person, please purchase an additional copy for each recipient. If you're reading this book and did not purchase it, or it was not purchased for your use only, then please return to your favourite retailer and purchase your own copy.

Thank you for respecting the hard work of this author.

First published as an eBook December 2021
First published in print November 2025
Special thanks to Tom McDermott,
for the cover design

Table of Contents

Why Makarasana

The Magic Briefly

How to Do Makarasana

Magic of Makarasana Videos and Audio links

A Deeper Understanding - Physical and Mental Benefits

A Deeper Understanding - Subtle Energy, Chakra and Emotional Benefits

Taking your Exploration Further - Connect with Teresa

About the Author

Why Makarasana

If there was one Yoga posture I would teach every single person in the world, knowing its power to transform, it would be Makarasana, also known as the Crocodile.

When practiced regularly and with awareness Makarasana brings peace and clarity into your life. It enables you to navigate stressful situations and builds resilience to stress and negativity. You find the capacity to heal and release negative emotions and return to a state of balance and harmony, allowing your natural state of happiness to bubble up from deep inside of you. It opens your heart to love, compassion and forgiveness, enabling self-acceptance, self-confidence and enhanced self-esteem.

Mentally you learn to detach from thoughts that don't serve you, to change your perception, see things differently and realise you have choices. These choices can set you free from the past and create a positive new future. You learn to connect with an inner strength, calm and a clarity that enables you to see and understand the truth of any situation. It builds courage and a strong will infused with determination.

Physically Makarasana aids many back, hip and shoulder issues, grounds your energy and infuses your whole being with vibrant health and well-being. Your body is nourished through deep relaxation that releases tension and fatigue, and the restoration of healthy sleep.

Spiritually you connect with the essence of who you are and find the source of life's magic.

This is why I believe whole heartedly that if everyone spent time in this amazing posture, the world would truly benefit. People would be happier, healthier and able to manage negative emotions and conflict so that living in peace and harmony would become a reality, not just a dream.

How can one Yoga posture

create so much Positive Change?

This is the reason I felt compelled to write this book, as over the past 20 years of teaching Dru Yoga I have explored this posture in depth and taught it to hundreds of people and seen the positive results in their lives. I feel passionate about sharing this with as many people as possible, both the science behind its many benefits as well as my own intuitive understanding and positive experience of this awesome technique.

Makarasana is named after the Makara, a crocodile like sea creature from Hindu Philosophy who guards thresholds and gateways to places of spiritual worship and wisdom. The Makara or crocodile moves easily between the land and the water thriving in both environments. Symbolically the land equates to our mind and the water to our emotions. This gives a hint at the power of our mind to see the truth and lift us up out of the waters of our emotional desire nature, least we drown in these waters. In flowing or moving easily between the two environments, Makarasana bridges and creates a connection between the heart and the mind allowing us to benefit from the wisdom of both working synergistically together. The ease with which the Makara moves teaches us that the key to opening this gate is to allow the emotions to flow, as in doing so they cleanse and heal our heart. By holding onto these emotions, we become stuck and unable to move forward, creating barriers to the natural flow of love from our heart.

This in turn affects the flow of our subtle energy and our vitality. When we are overwhelmed by strong emotion, feel stuck or blocked, this is when we need the Crocodile posture the most; not just to allow the emotions to flow in a way that is safe and healing but also to open the door to the understanding and insights in our mind we can gain as a result of experiencing those emotions. As a keeper of the gate, the Makara within us will allow the insights and understandings that we need to be revealed as and when we are ready for them. I will explore an understanding of the flow of subtle energy, and our chakra energy centres in relation to Makarasana later in this book.

Makarasana is simple to do

You don't have to be super fit or flexible

to spend time in Makarasana

Most people can practice it easily. It requires only 5-10minutes to make a profound difference and completely change how you are, what I call your whole state of 'Being'. If you can lie comfortably on your front on the floor you can do Makarasana. Even if you can't do this right away or for very long there are plenty of ways to modify this posture so that you can still gain the benefits.

One of the wonderful things about Yoga that never ceases to amaze is its power to affect us on all levels. It is a tradition that has evolved over thousands of years and still serves us now.

Every yoga position that we adopt has physical, energetic, emotional, mental and spiritual benefits with an extra magic that comes when you experience all these benefits together in the same moment.

Yoga means 'Union', and it is this power to bring about a complete union of all the different aspects of 'You' that creates the profound sense of well-being, deep healing and peace you experience when you practice yoga.

Practising just one Yoga posture, Makarasana will enable you to connect with the 'essence' or 'truth' of who you are and come to realise you are more complex, more powerful and have more control over how you feel and act in any given moment than you realise. It enables you to become incredibly resilient to life's ups and downs. You realise that no person or event in the world has the power to throw you off balance if you remain connected to something deep inside of you that is always strong, calm and clear, your inner balance.

Makarasana gives you an opportunity to retreat from life's dramas whenever you need to reconnect with your core or seek inner guidance to help navigate life's daily challenges. As you develop this 'union within' you enhance your capacity to develop heartfelt connections and come into union with others, and ultimately into union and peace with the world. You become less reactive and over time, more peaceful, proactive and positive in all areas of your life.

The magic of Makarasana is this capacity to reveal and connect you to the calm, clear, strong essence at the heart of each of us. This connection with your 'True Self' is only possible when you take some time to retreat from the busy outer world of the senses and take your awareness inward. From this place of stillness, you can experience rejuvenating peace and open to a surety about who you are and what is important and what actions you need to take. This cannot be adequately described in words but must be experienced.

I love to witness the change in people I teach when they spend time in this gentle yoga posture. They arise with a smile on their face, a twinkle in their eyes, they look younger, more peaceful and as if a huge burden has lifted. That smile that comes from their soul is why I love to teach yoga and meditation.

With regular practice of this wonderful posture, you come to see things differently, to gradually let go the hold of your ego and its filters through which you view the world and see truth instead. Our ego is that part of our mind that protects our view of our self, our perception of how things are and resists any change, growth or development of our understanding. As the ego loses its power you open to changing mental and emotional habits that no longer serve you. You have more choice about how you respond to other people and situations in your life, especially the challenging ones.

You naturally become more loving and accepting as you become more self-loving and self-accepting. This change is gentle and often something that other people will notice as enhanced confidence and joy. You will start to radiate vitality like you did as a child. Children have amazing adaptability and resilience, naturally accepting that they are growing and changing. In fact, they often enjoy new things, challenges, opportunities, finding change exciting.

If you feel you have lost this childlike wonder and desire to explore who you are, Makarasana will invite it to return.

As you welcome Makarasana into your life you will naturally develop greater conscious awareness and become more self-aware. You will see yourself differently, all your amazing attributes, as well as the areas in your development that need attention. You find the courage to look in the mirror, and smile with love at the awesome person you see, while seeking and inviting positive change.

This enhanced self-awareness triggers a natural healing process and a trust in the wisdom that is found within you to intuitively guide you through this journey. As you learn to let go of who you are not, you will find it easier to express who you are, to be creative, spontaneous allowing your light to shine out into the world. This brings a wonderful sense of freedom, is deeply fulfilling and will help those around you. When you have the courage to show up in life as your authentic 'Self' you unconsciously give others permission to do the same and they feel at ease around you.

This light is who you are, your 'True Self', not a false ego self that craves love, approval or attention, fears rejection from others, fears judgement and criticism. Rather a sense of self that is happy, joyful and simply 'is'. You come to stand in 'All That You Are' and know that this is awesome. This transformation is the magic of the Crocodile and something that is waiting for you if you want it....

I think of yoga and meditation as tools you add to your toolkit to cope with life. Makarasana is one of the most important of these tools. Its power is its inherent ability to bring you back to feeling strong, calm and clear whenever life throws you challenges that knock you off balance and to understand what caused your response. You have the perfect way to return to peace and harmony with a clear mind, connected to your hearts intelligence and a chance to be open to solutions that were not previously assessable.

Often, we are aware of what needs healing within us, but we don't know what to do about it. We don't know **how** to begin, and we feel trapped in a cycle of almost automatic, unconscious behaviour patterns that we really want to change. Makarasana gives you a very practical way to begin the releasing and healing process. This is why it is such a valuable tool. It teaches us how to change.

I want to share just how powerful this posture is from my own experience.

I am familiar with life throwing me off balance, as a single mother of four children, there have been times when I have felt stuck, not knowing how to move forward, feeling exhausted, overwhelmed and that a situation is hopeless.

But I know that if I simply spend time in Makarasana, breathe, relax and connect with my true Self the situation comes into perspective. My body calms down, strong emotions release, and this gives me a chance to see and let go the negative thought loops I recognise are not helping me.

These patterns are often quite familiar to us when we step back and observe them in this way. Makarasana will naturally develop this capacity for greater self-reflection and enhance your self-awareness and capacity to witness your thoughts and emotions in a detached way.

It does require honesty and a commitment to be lovingly kind with your-self as you heal and grow. Many people avoid facing truths about themself from a fear of what they might discover; that deep down they are not good enough or worthy of love.

They believe it is easier to look for fulfilment and happiness in the things and experiences of the world than believing that these qualities can be found by looking within themselves. They will avoid self-evaluation and self-discovery as they associate it with judgement and criticism. In my experience it is quite the opposite when you connect with the essence within you. This feeling of connection affirms you are loved and cherished unconditionally, beyond measure, from the part of you that knows the truth of all that you are, including those aspects that still need healing. The more you do Makarasana the more this loving kind relationship with your true Self develops and the easier and safer it becomes to be brutally honest with yourself. It eventually becomes your natural way of being. As your honest connection with yourself grows you find that your relationships with others reflect this honesty, openness and authenticity.

By coming into Makarasana I am willing to surrender the situation to something wiser than my usual thought processes and ask for help. I would describe this as surrendering my ego's desire to be right and hold onto my current perspective. Sometimes this resistance manifests as avoidance tactics and I will find reasons not to do Makarasana. This is because part of me wants to hold onto the anger, the sense of injustice and grievance for longer. But eventually the part of me that wants to heal prompts me and I just get down on the floor and surrender because I know from my experience that this always results in a positive transformation.

I experience this as the magic that allows wonderful realisations and understandings about the situation to flow into my awareness. Often there are tears as I realise what is going on at a deeper level, the truth from my Soul's perspective. I see my time in Makarasana like time in meditation, it is spending time with my Highest Self or Soul connecting me to my inner wisdom and allowing a conversation about what is troubling me, perplexing me or simply overwhelming me. The tension leaves my body, and I can relax and breathe again. My curiosity arises as I seek to understand the situation.

> **'There is no greater battle, than the battle between the parts of you that want to be healed and the parts of you that are comfortable and content remaining broken'**
>
> Author unknown

Ancient wisdom teachings assure us that the wise part of us, our Soul or Higher Self always has our best interests at heart and wants us to grow, evolve and step into the best version of who we are. This is to become more consciously aware. It is the development of this awareness that activates the healing response from our deepest Self. But we need to seek this guidance and step out of life for a few moments and have the courage to go within.

When we are too busy thinking, our conscious mind gets caught up and totally focused on our thoughts. By developing our capacity to bring our mind into connection with our inner stillness we can step back from our thoughts and allow the voice of our inner wisdom to be heard.

Once I have relaxed and connected with the peace within me, I will see the reason for what is going on and how the challenges are giving me the opportunity to develop strengths and capacities that I didn't have before. I feel empowered.

As these realisations flow, I find courage and often excitement bubbles up within me as I start to open to a new way of seeing the situation and this brings the most amazing solutions. Sometimes these come complete, whole and take my breath away with their perfection. These are the 'aha' moments we can experience when we let go and simply open to new possibilities.

But often I come to see my part in the drama, the parts of me that still need healing, that were triggered, and I realise that the other person was doing the best they could with all that needs healing in them. This brings me to the peace of acceptance, and often to forgiveness, compassion and understanding. I can let go the situation, the issue, the grievance or whatever threw me off balance and return to peace.

'Awareness is like the sun.

When it shines on things they are transformed'

Thich Nhat Hanh

I have explored a deeper understanding of forgiveness for years and found that many people have the mistaken belief that acceptance, compassion and forgiveness are qualities that we bestow on others. Through this process of surrender in Makarasana we come to realise that these are gifts we give our self.

To forgive another you don't have to involve them at all, it does not condone their behaviour but sets you free from your response to that behaviour. Forgiveness is all about what you are holding on to, and the negative effect it is having on you, and this is attachment at the level of the ego.

We are not responsible for the behaviour

of other people,

We are only ever responsible for our own behaviour

By letting go of our anger, our resentment, our story we can be free of these health destroying emotions and create a space. This space gives us the freedom to choose. From this place of freedom, you have options and choices about what you might or might not do about this situation. You may intuitively feel you don't need to do anything. Releasing the resentment and anger and returning to love and acceptance was all the healing that was required. If you need to have a calm, honest, loving conversation with another about the issue you can do so without the toxic emotions. By approaching another from a place of empowerment and compassion there is an increased likelihood that a change for the better can take place. You will be able to preserve the connection or union with that person you care about while still solving a problem that has arisen. Sometimes the other person is not ready to take responsibility for their part, move forward and let go and in this case, you simply need to practice accepting what is and trust in the Universe to bring about the necessary change and healing in time. You may choose to simply walk away at this time.

The key to understanding this process is realising that it is the energy of anger, upset or grief that needs to release so that a resolution can be found. When we become overwhelmed by the need to release this energy of strong emotions that have been triggered, this is when we fall back into reactive patterns of behaviour. We literally explode with the need to release this energy. Makarasana offers a gentle private personal way to release the energy so that you can then address the issue with a calm mind and open-hearted intention to resolve what needs healing.

This whole experience is such a gift, and I am so profoundly grateful for the process. The magic is a power inherent in this simple yoga posture, Makarasana that gives you the choice to remain peaceful and return to this state of peace whenever life disturbs your peace.

I have found that by choosing to go into Makarasana whenever I am upset or angry or out of sorts or just need some time to myself to recharge, I am taking responsibility for how I am feeling and deciding to honour myself and the situation by doing something positive about it. It sets me free and everyone else involved free of the potential damage of holding grievances, injustices and resentments that damage relationships. Everyone involved can return to peace, health and love. Holding onto this negative energy is exhausting and can ultimately damage our health as I will explore later in this book. When we come back to place of connection and union with our Self, we keep the door open to continuing connection and unity with others. Choosing this process of inner transformation is how we change our world and our experience of our life. This choice to respond differently empowers us and this in turn empowers others. Through our own personal process of growth and positive change we make a difference in the world.

In my experience my children or anyone I am relating to, benefit as I can be a better mum, a better person and create an environment that is a happier, and more peaceful. By taking responsibility for how I am I can create a safe haven where it is ok to feel strong emotions, but I teach by example that it is the responsibility of each of us to deal with our reactions and return to peace and then address any issues that need resolving from this place of understanding. This is the seeds of emotional intelligence that we teach best by example.

The beauty is that without saying a word by simply practising Makarasana, I am teaching those I care about how to deal with their strong reactions to life and a way to return to peace whenever life throws them off balance.

I certainly don't always get it right and often need to work on a particular issue over a period. From experience I know that any new skill takes time to learn and master, but patience and perseverance will always bring healing and a positive breakthrough. By practising loving kindness with my Self, I create an environment of acceptance and a way of living that is heart centred. This acceptance of my own humanness, my frailty and my imperfections extends to everyone around me, so that the process of growth and change becomes safe and welcome in my home. Spiritual growth is fostered and nurtured even if this is not spoken of or recognised.

When you make the choice to do Makarasana you don't just do this posture for your own benefit, but you do it for everyone you care about.

In recounting my experience of Makarasana I have simply given you a taste of the emotional, and mind changing potential of this posture. There are numerous physical, energetic and spiritual benefits that I will reveal as we continue this journey of exploration into the magic of the Crocodile.

> **'Only one who devotes himself to a cause with his whole strength and soul can be a true master. For this reason, mastery demands all of a person'**
>
> Albert Einstein

Makarasana is a master posture. In the yoga tradition a posture is only deemed a master posture when it has profound benefits on all levels of your being to return you to inner peace, harmony and alignment. I have seen Makarasana transform the whole demeanour of teenagers, bring peace and emotional calm to autistic children and tears to the eyes of their parents, cure insomnia and gently augment deep healing and release in clients who have experienced major trauma, grief, or upset. It is used to bring peace, forgiveness and understanding to those living in constant conflict in war zones.

Its power is something you can only really appreciate when you witness it first-hand. I remember years ago, a mother coming up to me in the playground at my local primary school as we were waiting to collect our younger children and ask me what I had done to her teenage daughter. I had taken a very short 15minute relaxation at the local High School that day and encouraged the students to do it in Makarasana. She had tears in her eyes as she said her daughter had come home peaceful and happy. They had a nice conversation and that was the best she had seen and experienced from her daughter in years.

This posture is Magic!!

I am only aware of two other master postures, Tadasana, The Mountain Posture and Nataraj asana, The Dancer. These are subjects for further books but if you want to know more for now, visit www.teresa4yoga.co.uk or go to my YouTube channel Teresa Keast and search: Teresa teaching Tadasana the Mountain Posture with Deep Yogic Breathing, to watch a 10-

minute video in which I teach you how to do Tadasana and breathe for health, calm and vitality.

Now that I have introduced you to Makarasana I will outline how I plan to take you deeper into both an experience of and an understanding of this marvellous posture.

I will start by briefly listing the benefits of Makarasana to give you a taste of its magic.

Then I will teach you how to practice Makarasana including links to YouTube videos you can watch and audio tracks you can download so that you can experience it for yourself, including any modifications needed so it is comfortable for everyone to do.

The rest of this book will be devoted to exploring each of the many benefits in much more depth, both from an ancient wisdom and a modern scientific viewpoint so that you can really understand what is happening when you choose to spend time in Makarasana.

It is my hope that this posture will ignite within you a desire to begin the process of healing that is the foundation of an authentic way of living. Through the process of surrender I trust you will come to embrace the benefits of this one yoga posture and perhaps this will lead you to explore yoga and perhaps meditation in more depth. I believe one of the profound keys to leading a happy and healthy life is to become aware of your life's purpose and give your existence meaning. Through yoga and meditation, I have come to realise the joy of finding my unique path in this life and sincerely wish this for everyone as it brings such joy, challenges, surrender and then more joy.

If you have never explored yoga before this is a perfect place to start. If you are a yoga convert, then I trust this posture will add further dimension to your love and understanding of this profound practice.

Approach with an open mind and heart and let's see where the magic takes you….

After reading this information I am confident you will want to practice the Crocodile regularly and to teach everyone you know this fabulous technique and together we can start teaching the world.

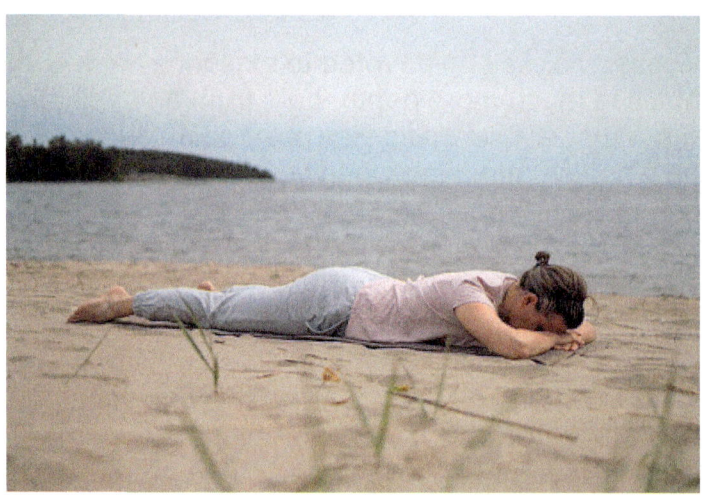

The Magic Briefly

'Hitch your Wagon to a Star'

Ralph Waldo Emerson

- Enhances Diaphragmatic or Deep Belly breathing, with its numerous health benefits
- Improves many impaired breathing conditions or poor inefficient breathing
- Detoxifies the physical body, improves lymph flow and promotes a healthy immune system
- Improves digestive function and relieves many digestive complaints
- Reduces shoulder, neck and back tension
- Opens the chest area and improves posture of the upper body, this is especially beneficial for those who sit a lot and tend to slouch
- Physically good for relieving slipped disc, sciatica, lower back pain or other spinal disorders
- Improves your posture
- Evokes the deep 'Relaxation response' in your body, releasing tension and fatigue, reducing stress and building resilience to the negative effects of stress mentally, emotionally and physically

- Grounds your energy and opens the base chakra connecting you with the energy of the Earth and the health benefits this brings

- Clears your mind and brings you to a place of peace in your mind

- Allows you to experience simply 'Being' and restores your harmony and equilibrium

- Cultivates present moment awareness and mindfulness

- Brings a balance between 'being' and 'doing' in your everyday life

- Brings the yin, feminine, left side of your body into balance with the yang, masculine, right side of your body and allows you to return to peace and harmony within yourself and in your life

- Helps to restore hormonal balance especially in times of hormonal change

- Calms the nervous system and builds vagal nerve tone that builds resilience to stress and the negative effects of external conditions in your life

- Helps to restore the natural cycles in your body, sleeping and waking, energy peaks and troughs

- Restores your vitality by allowing more Prana or Chi to come into and flow through the subtle energy channels in your body

- Encourages the flow of energy between the major energy centres/chakras, and flow from the lower chakras to the higher chakras

- Recalibrates your whole vitality and subtle energy system

- Connects your head intelligence to your heart intelligence to help with decision making and resolving inner conflicts

- Develops Heart Coherence and all its positive health benefits

- Brings you into alignment with your inner intuitive wisdom through your third eye or Ajna chakra

- Opens the Anahata, Heart chakra, developing trust, courage and the capacity to forgive, give and receive love and live from a place of gratitude

- Facilitates emotional release of strong emotional energy, like anger, jealousy, pride, fear, doubt, anxiety, upset, grief or irritation

- Gently releases trauma from the tissues

- Returns you to peace emotionally and understanding mentally

- Brings insights into conflicts and aids resolution, understanding, acceptance and ultimately forgiveness

- Can help to alleviate and manage anxiety attacks and works overtime to allow the release of the emotional causes of depression

- Releases emotionally generated back and neck tension

- Connects your conscious mind with your hidden unconscious mind bringing understanding, healing and positive transformation

- Enhances self-awareness, self-honesty and reflection
- Improves insomnia and promotes better quality sleep and dreams
- Takes the benefits of other yoga postures deeper
- Perfect for starting or finishing the day feeling peaceful and calm, or for naturally moving into meditation
- Improves the flow of creative energy, including sexual energy and its healthy expression
- Empowers a life of purpose and meaning
- Restores your Inner Joy!!
- Is Relaxing and calming especially done outside in nature

How to Do Makarasana

'Quality is not an act; it is a habit'

Aristotle

Makarasana is often used as a relaxation yoga posture and one of the best poses for facilitating diaphragmatic or Deep Yogic Breathing.

It is not recommended after the first 3 months of pregnancy or during pregnancy when lying on your front is uncomfortable and may not be comfortable whilst breastfeeding or for several months after abdominal surgery.

While Makarasana helps to improve the strength of the diaphragm and aids many people with compromised breathing or breathing disorders it is not recommended if you feel undue constriction in the chest while in the posture. See possible modifications later in this book.

At first there might be some discomfort especially if your body is tight across the shoulders, upper back, chest or neck so it would be advisable to simply stay in the posture for a short time and gradually increase that time as your body adapts and the tension eases.

Makarasana is contraindicated if the posture causes any discomfort in your back, especially if you have had any recent spinal injuries or problems. For most people it eases lower back pain and aids recovery from slipped disc, sciatica, and other spinal disorders. It can relieve the downward pressure on spinal discs and help to reduce compression of spinal nerves. It eases general back stiffness.

But you must listen to your body and work within your own comfort zone. Remember pain is the body's way of telling you something isn't right. If in doubt as to whether the posture is suitable for you, please check with your medical practitioner.

'The Secret of getting ahead is getting started'

Mark Twain

So let us begin…

I would advise reading through these instructions, including the possible modifications you can use to improve your comfort whilst in Makarasana.

At the end of this section, you will find information about a video in which I guide you into Makarasana, the Crocodile posture and teach these modifications.

You will also find two Guided Relaxations specifically designed to use with your practice of Makarasana.

The first focuses primarily on Relaxing and simply 'Being' in the posture for 10 minutes.

The second is 20 minutes long and gives you the opportunity to go into a meditative state to access your inner intuitive guidance and release negative emotions.

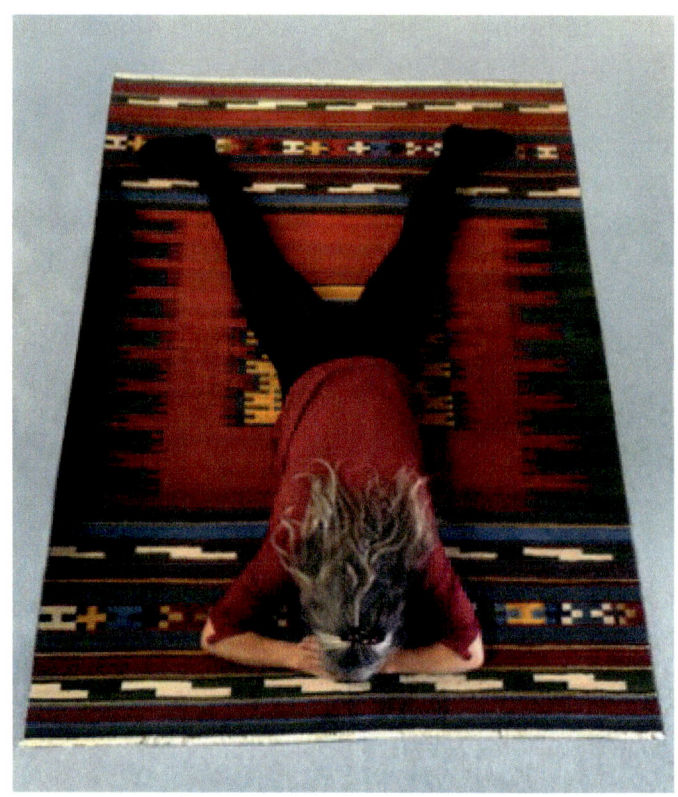

The Author in Makarasana

This is your time to deeply relax, heal and rejuvenate

Find a place where you will not be disturbed and you feel you can relax, ideally where you can lie on the floor on carpet or a rug, a yoga mat or blanket. Turn off your phone and any other distractions. You may find it helpful to create a nice atmosphere, burn some incense, dim any strong light or play some gentle relaxing music softly. Ensure you are warm enough and there is adequate ventilation in the room.

Ideally set aside ten minutes, although if you have been very upset or are seeking specific guidance or inner counsel to resolve an issue you may need to spend longer.

To come into Makarasana stretch out on the floor, face down with your legs reasonably straight, relaxed and comfortably spread apart. Ideally turn your toes outward and your heels inward. Place one hand on top of the other, palms facing down, with your elbows extended to the sides while you rest your forehead on your hands.

See if you can relax in this position especially across the upper back, the hips and pelvis. If this is not comfortable for your head or your neck and shoulders you can fold your arms and place your hands on opposite elbows. Lower your head and rest your forehead on your forearms. Or cross your arms, bringing your hands to your opposite shoulders, and rest your forehead on your arms.

The important thing is that you can relax across the shoulders and between the shoulder blades and back of your neck and allow your abdomen to rest fully on the floor. There will be a slight feeling of elevation in your upper chest.

Relax your pelvis and hips and imagine that they are continuing to release into the floor as you settle into the posture.

Relax through your feet and ankles allowing your legs to release into the floor.

Close your eyes and relax your face, head, neck, shoulders, abdomen, pelvis, legs and feet and breathe gently. It is ideal to breathe through your nose if this is comfortable.

Possible modifications

If you don't find this position comfortable across your shoulders, upper back and neck, especially if resting in the posture for 5-10minutes, you can place a thin cushion or folded towel under your upper chest. This eases the tension in the shoulders and neck and allows you to breathe more easily through your nose.

If your forehead is uncomfortable place a towel, blanket or thin cushion on top of your hands and then rest your forehead.

It is important to be able to relax through the pelvis, hips and legs. If the position of your feet is uncomfortable with the toes turned out and the heels turned in, you can place cushions under each ankle until your flexibility improves and you find this position easier. Try taking your legs a bit further apart to release through the hips.

As you settle into the posture bring your attention to your breath. You will find that as you inhale your abdomen is naturally pressing into the floor or the mat and as you exhale there is a gentle release of this pressure. As you breathe in let there be a gentle feeling of expansion into your lower back with a flaring and expansion of the lower ribs. It helps to imagine that as you breathe in your body is opening and expanding and as you breathe out your body is relaxing down into the floor with a feeling of surrender or letting go.

Continue breathing slowly and deeply so that you feel your tummy press into the floor as you breathe in and as you breathe out you allow yourself to sink a little deeper into the floor.

If you notice that one side of your body feels different to the other side, perhaps lighter or heavier, tense or in spasm. Acknowledge this observation and then set an intention that during your practice your body will find its alignment, restoring balance and harmony and you will become aware of anything that is causing this imbalance, so that you can make the necessary changes in your life.

Keep your awareness gently on your breath and imagine as it comes in through your nose it travels down through a channel deep in your body between the sternum or breastbone and your spine all the way into your belly. Follow the course of your breath with your attention and your mind. Then as you breathe out you imagine your breath returns along this channel and releases out through your nose or your mouth. With each cycle this channel clears and opens and your body relaxes from deep inside, allowing this opening, expanding feeling to radiate out to all parts of your physical body. You relax from the inside, outward.

Keep breathing and relaxing and maintain a gentle focus on your breath and by keeping this focus you will allow your breath to take you into connection with a quiet space inside. This is a place of stillness in your mind where you feel calm, peaceful, strong and clear. You will find that your thoughts slow down and there is space between them.

 By gently focusing on the breath, you will be able to detach or step back from your thoughts and connect with your inner sanctuary. Whenever your mind becomes distracted by physical sensations, sounds or enticing thoughts, as soon as you realise you have been distracted, simply return to a gentle focus on the breath. Return with no feeling of judgement or criticism. This is **important** as the judgement and criticism are simply ego generated. Return to a focus on the breath with loving kindness and a gentle acceptance. It doesn't matter if your mind wanders, this is quite normal, what does matter is that you return to the breath with loving kindness. Imagine the breath is taking you by the hand and leading you deep into the stillness that is found within you. Your breath is the great connector between mind and body, and mind, body and soul. When you focus consciously on the breath you become aware of the union of these parts of your being.

Continue to rest in Makarasana simply breathing, relaxing and enjoying the feeling of just 'being' and having nothing you must do until you feel refreshed, recharged, balanced and peaceful again.

Releasing Whatever Arises

If during your practice you feel a tension building especially around the solar plexus or the chest area and a discomfort that might even feel a little panicky. First, just accept this and see if you can relax and give yourself permission to feel whatever it is and not push it away, opening to the idea that you could let it release. Sometimes this release will be quite physical, a feeling of energy moving up your body and out of your throat or the top of your head. But it will feel emotional, and you may find yourself crying or realise you want to cry, scream or shout. Just accept these feelings and breathe with them having the intention that the discomfort will release and set you free. Crying heals the heart; emotion is energy that needs to be in motion to exert its healing power.

It can be scary at first but if you can stay with that feeling just once, breathing deeply you will learn to release negative emotions in this way.

This is not something that will always happen or might not happen at all, but I want you to know that it is a perfectly natural part of the process of letting go old patterns of emotional energy, old beliefs and attitudes that no longer serve you and moving through this transformation to a new place where that energy has gone. Don't be frightened by this. It is a positive, purifying process. The secret is to surrender and trust the part of you that is wise and knows this release is for your highest good and part of your growth and healing and a transformation that is beautiful. The immense relief you will feel if you can find the courage to move through this release will be worth it.

It might take a few sessions in Makarasana if you have some strong emotions, traumas, or issues to release, as often we are quite resistant to this process until we have experienced just how good it feels when you have had the courage to move through the discomfort to the wonderful sense of well-being and peace that settles in your core after such a release. Trust me; the short-term discomfort is well worth the peace after the release and the lifetime of freedom from the pain of that issue and deeper insights into its causes and effects and potential redemption. But you need to develop a trust in this process yourself and that can take time. It will require patience and persistence.

Sometimes you will be conscious of what is releasing, an old memory may come up or something you thought you had healed presents itself in your mind. Don't dismiss anything, no matter how trivial it may appear. Our intuitive mind tends to communicate in symbols and feelings many people describe as gut feelings. Often your ego mind wants to discount valuable information before you have had the chance to register or contemplate the wisdom it might reveal. If your mind is analysing, discussing or having a conversation about the issue, this is the ego talking. Just ignore this tirade and come back to focusing on the breath and the feeling of allowing. Sometimes you will not be consciously aware of what has or needs to be released, so just let it go anyway, trusting that the wise intuitive part of you knows what is needed for your healing and growth.

I remember the first time I really understood the power of Makarasana. It was just after my marriage of 20 years had just broken up and I had been holding it all together, strong and calm for my four children, clear about what I had to do to sort out my life and help them through the changes. I thought I was doing fine and dealing with it all. Then I came into this wonderful posture and the flood gates opened and I sobbed with such raw relief and let go so much emotional energy, the hopes and dreams, the frustrations and uncertainties, the anger and upset. Luckily, I was on the last weekend of my yoga training and surrounded by people who totally understood what I was experiencing and welcomed my surrender. The incredible relief I felt afterwards was awesome. I felt like I had been washed clean, and I felt truly strong and clear and a sense that I could rise to this challenge and my life would be better. I knew intuitively it was for the good of all and the right decision and I felt empowered and knew I could help my kids come through this challenge. I knew it was important to show them how to navigate these new waters and be bold and rise above the fears and doubts and embrace the changes positively.

There were so many things I understood and gained instant clarity on that I had to go and write them down. But most of all I realised that I had just taken the first steps on a new path and that this path was the right one for me. My marriage breakup was a positive thing that in time I would see as a major turning point in my spiritual life.

I was exhausted and needed sleep to recover but felt like in a short space of time I had already moved significantly forward. I was in awe of this posture from that moment on.

I have helped many clients and yoga students release significant traumas and hurt from the past in this way and afterwards they have been tearful with relief and gratitude for the gift of Makarasana. Sometimes it helps to have someone you trust with you, just to place a hand on your back or your shoulder supporting you unconditionally without judgement. Some people prefer to be on their own during this process of release.

The following is a list of symptoms and experiences that we commonly experience when there is something that needs to release.

- Feeling at odds with life
- Tense for no obvious reason
- Feeling like something needs or is about to happen or a growing tension
- Feeling angry, frustrated and reactive or over-reacting to situations
- Feeling weepy or sad for no obvious reason
- Feeling physical tension or a blocked bloated heavy feeling around the centre of your torso, especially in your solar plexus or in your gut
- Feeling a tightness around the centre of your chest, or that something is pressing down on your chest
- A continual need to clear your throat, or feeling like words or emotions are stuck in your throat

- Unexplained fatigue and lethargy, a loss of purpose and joy
- Unexplained aches and pains and general feeling you are not right
- Waking in the wee small hours unable to get back to sleep

Over the years I have found if you have something you know needs to release but there is a resistance to letting it go, answering the following statements while in Makarasana, with total honestly from your heart can help spark the process of release.

In my experience, these words get to the core of the resistance and trapped emotional issues have shifted quite quickly after I have repeated them from my heart with conviction and honesty. But recognise that this is something that takes practice and some time for you to trust. Give it a go and see how it feels for you…

Can I let this go?

Will I let this go?

When?

Don't despair if whatever is creating the aggravation within you doesn't release the first time you try. It may have been there for a very long time and often relates to childhood experiences or traumas that you fear as you don't want to revisit the pain.

Sometimes you can be frightened by the intensity of your feelings and wary of what might happen if you express this built-up emotional energy. There can be concern that you will be totally out of control.

Be assured, you don't have to experience the full pain at all, there is some grief, and it is not necessarily pleasant during the release but nothing like the pain of the original episode. You will feel an instant relief from the tension that was created by holding onto the negative energy associated with this situation and the tears that often follow are healing tears, not tears of despair and frustration. It's what I call 'good crying'.

I find it helps to think of me now as an emotionally mature adult going back in time and being the wise supportive person I needed back then, who just holds the damaged child within me and allows her to let go her pain safely because I understand and I am there for her unconditionally. Once your inner child has released the hurt, grief and emotional traumas you can imagine bringing him/her into your heart now, healed and restored. This can be a powerful visualisation to augment release and healing.

Accessing Intuitive Wisdom

If you choose to spend a little longer in The Crocodile and focus on the breath allowing your mind to quieten down to connect with the peaceful, stillness within you, there is the opportunity to go deeper into this meditative state and access your higher states of awareness and intuitive wisdom.

From this place of deep connection, you can simply ask the questions you seek answers to in your life at any given time. Or if you are not sure of the questions but just have a vague sense of unease and restlessness you can ask….

What do I need right here, right now?

Then simply be completely open, impartial and unattached to any particular outcome or result so that you don't distort or block the process.

See what comes into your awareness.

The key is to be completely relaxed and centred within yourself, so that you can maintain a deep connection to your intuitive wisdom.

Like most new skills this will require practice to master, so be patient and persevere, giving yourself time to determine how valid an inner prompting may be before you decide to act on it. This requires discernment and will naturally develop your discrimination. With practice you will come to recognise the unique way your wise Soul or Higher Self communicates with you. This 'higher' aspect of you is in direct communication with the Universal field of wisdom, or infinite knowledge far beyond that which our minds can determine and we can tap into this through deep meditative states. The inner prompting, insights and understanding that arise are always just exactly what you need in any given moment in time. The key is to have the courage to seek and trust this wisdom.

Guidance seldom arrives in words and is more often symbolic, particularly meaningful to you, a feeling about a situation or a pull in a certain direction. It might involve a flashback memory or a sudden realisation or knowing. This 'knowing' is something you feel to be irrefutable and right even if you can't explain or understand why. It just 'is' and has a quality unlike any usual thought derived through analysis or pondering. Often it arises spontaneously and is beautiful in its simplicity and the way it solves all problems, synergises all understanding and transports you instantly to a new level of insight and inspiration.

I have had the experience that when seeking the answer to a question a particular song kept popping into my mind and when I eventually listened to the words, they were exactly what I needed. I cried with the beauty of it.

Sometimes the answers will come in dreams that night or over the next few nights or a recurring memory when you are in a daydreaming state.

If you can remain open and aware, with an attitude of curiosity, you will be surprised by the seemingly miraculous. Someone will say just what you needed to hear, or you will receive an email, or some other coincidence will occur in your life, and you will recognise the answer to your question. I always give thanks to my Higher Self and its connection to the Universe and smile when these serendipitous moments occur. But be assured that when you genuinely ask, the answers always come to you in some way. Sometimes we miss them when we are not paying attention. So, remain open and curious with an expectation of miracles. This is where a practice of mindfulness, remaining centred in the present moment, not caught up in thoughts that stem from the past or ruminating about the future is of immense benefit to ensuring you don't miss these 'pearls of wisdom'.

To explore more about Meditation and Intuition visit my website teresa4yoga.co.uk or you can search YouTube Teresa Keast meditation and intuition where there are several videos or read an article on my Substack page teresakeast.substack.com

My Magic of Makarasana Twenty-minute Guided Relaxation on YouTube is designed for deeper relaxation and healing and to allow you to release any strong emotions or emotional issues that arise. It will allow you to dive deeper into a meditative state to access your intuitive wisdom. I would highly recommend spending an extended time in this posture at least once a week or as your need arises.

Take your time coming out of the posture. Bring your feet together, place your hands under your shoulders and roll onto your right side and rest for a moment supporting your head before you slowly sit up. Alternatively, you might want to stretch out your back in the extended child with your knees apart before you slowly come up.

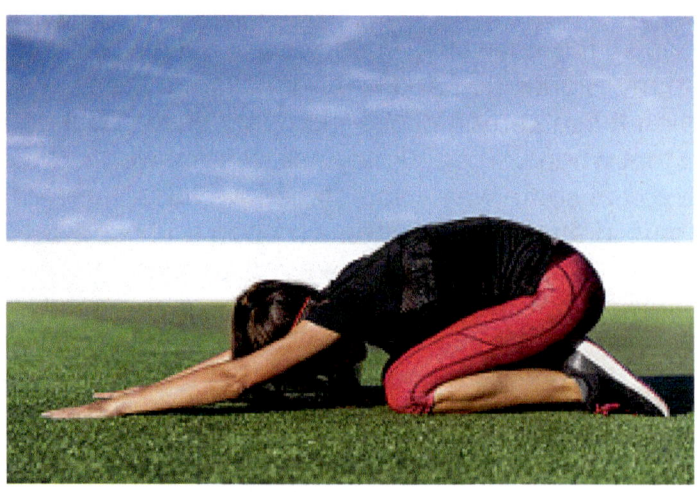

Ensure you drink plenty of water, or any liquid that doesn't contain alcohol, caffeine, sugar or sweeteners. Aim to drink at least one and up to two litres over the couple of hours following a longer session in Makarasana. Ideally take small sips often. This helps with the energetic, emotional and physical detox and healing process of this amazing posture.

Take it easy for a while after a longer practice of Makarasana. If you feel a little lightheaded it might pay to ground your energy by going outside in nature and just sitting and breathing or walking barefoot on the ground or even better on wet grass or paddling in a river or the sea. If this is not possible you can use the following very effective Qi Gong exercise.

Qi gong exercise to Ground your energy

Standing or sitting take your awareness to your feet. Gently close your eyes.

Imagine you are breathing in through gaps under your toes, breathe along the sole of your foot and breathe out through a gap in your heels.

The energy is coming up from the earth, along your foot and returning to the earth in a cycle. Repeat this breathing visualisation for nine breath cycles, breathing at a pace and depth that feels natural and comfortable for you. You know you are grounded when you open your eyes, and your head has cleared, and your feet feel like you are wearing lead boots and are very definitely connected to the earth and what is important.

Magic of Makarasana Video and Audios

You can find the following videos on my YouTube channel 'Teresa Keast' that teach you how to do Makarasana including possible modifications and separate guided relaxations to listen to as you relax in Makarasana, with or without background music.

Magic of Makarasana, how to do the Crocodile Yoga Posture with Teresa

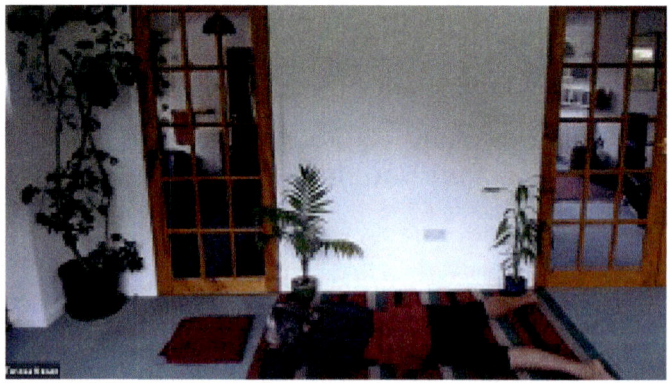

Teresa's Magic of Makarasana Ten minute

Guided Relaxation

(one with background music and another without)

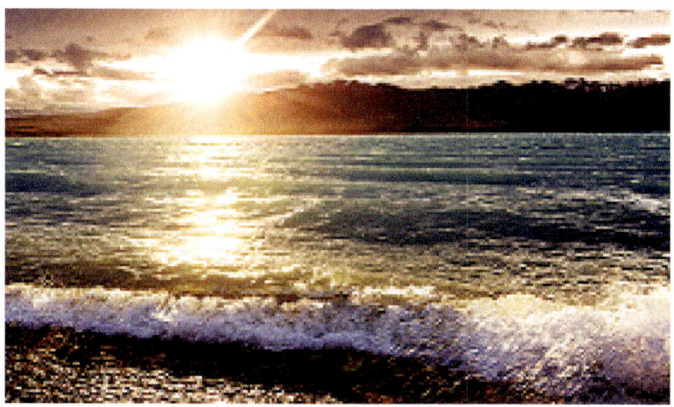

Teresa's Magic of Makarasana Twenty minute

Guided Relaxation (no background music)

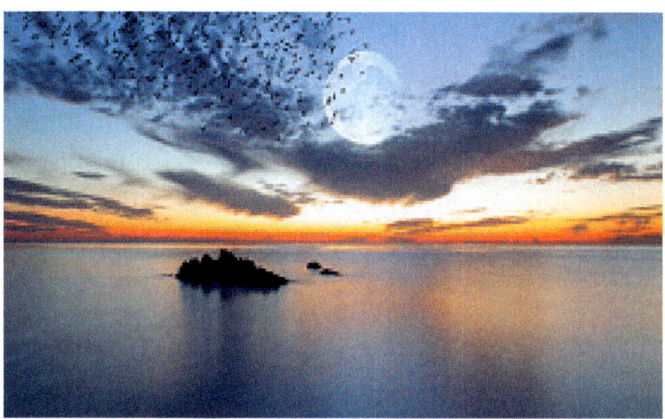

A Deeper Understanding

Physical and Mental Benefits

Physically the Crocodile helps to open your pelvis and release tension in the muscles in and around your lower back and hips, improving flexibility and your range of movement. Over time it will ease lower back ache and sacro-iliac joint issues if there is no underlying structural misalignment. It can release inflexibility in the muscles, tendons and ligaments around the knees and enhance ankle flexibility. You will find enhanced flexibility in the adductor muscles in the inside thigh. When these are particularly tight this can compromise the healthy function of both the knee and hip joint. Makarasana will also help to stretch and release the hip flexor muscles at the front of your hips. Tight hip flexors can create a tilt in your pelvis and alter your posture so that there is increased strain on your lower back. Hip flexors and hamstrings tend to tighten when we sit a lot potentially contributing to lower back discomfort.

Makarasana helps to release the tension that builds especially in the top of your shoulders and between your shoulder blades. As the muscles in this area release, lengthen and relax, the chest and upper back can open and expand and there is a subsequent release in tension through the shoulder joints and up into the neck and back of the head. This greatly improves your posture especially if you tend to round your shoulders or spend a lot of time working at a computer or driving. The release in tension can relieve chronic headaches and problems with concentration as it enhances the blood circulation through the neck and head to the brain. The opening of your chest will also improve the capacity and efficiency of your breathing.

We all have habits of posture and areas of our body where we carry tension. You may have noticed that when you start to feel stressed your neck and shoulders tighten, your chest constricts, and it feels as if a band of tension is wrapping around your ribcage in both the front and back of your body that stops you breathing fully and deeply. Some people find their jaw tightens, or they experience a knot in their stomach. We are all unique in the exact pattern that we habitually adopt in response to certain stressful, worrying, or anxious thoughts but the beauty of spending time in Makarasana is that you can slowly and surely change your body's habitual posture and these patterns of holding tension. This change naturally occurs through regular practice of this wonderful posture and is enhanced through the release of mental and emotional tension that the Crocodile allows. You literally relax into a new way of being physically, mentally and emotionally. I will talk more about the mental and emotional benefits later in this book.

As you practice Makarasana there will be a gradual release of the habitual tension we often carry in and around the mid and lower back and a release of the tendency of your ribs to contract down into your hips. This allows your natural waist to return and creates a lengthening through your torso and a corresponding space inside. In effect your body will begin to open and expand giving more space for optimal organ function, circulation, immune function and subsequent health. Tense muscles use a lot of energy, so as you relax this energy is available for your daily life. There is also a powerful effect on the flow of subtle energy which you experience as vitality in your body, which I will talk about later in this book.

The elongated position of your body with your heels turned out and toes turned inward helps to lengthen the fascia connective tissue network throughout your body. Recent studies are finding many positive benefits of keeping your fascia stretched and activated in this way that prevent age related stiffness in this connective tissue. We used to think fascia was inert and simply wrapped around muscles and organs to keep them in place structurally, but now we know it plays a vital part in the whole communication network in your physical body and when stretched regularly can positively interact to change the biochemistry and physiology of the body systems it supports. The wonderful thing about stretching your whole body in this way is that it activates chains of fascia that link throughout your body so that you experience the benefits from the top of your head to the tip of your toes.

Health Enhancing Diaphragmatic or Deep Yogic Breathing

Makarasana is one of the best Yoga postures to develop what we call diaphragmatic breathing or Deep Yogic Breathing

This is a natural health promoting way of breathing into your belly, taking the breath deeper and slowing it down.

If you watch the way small babies breathe you will notice that as they breathe in their tummy rises and as they breathe out their tummy falls and the chest and collar bones simply follow this full body movement. This is the way we were designed to breathe and the best technique for optimal health. I will now explore this in more detail.

Most people don't breathe properly, they chest breathe, so that when they breathe in their chest rises filling with air and when they breathe out the chest lowers back again. Chest breathing overuses the muscles of the neck and shoulders and can create chronic muscle tension and pain in this area. As the diaphragm muscle is not being used it can become weak and less effective.

This way of breathing is simply a habit that you often learned from about the age of 2 years old when you copied how your parents breathed as part of a naturally built in survival mechanism to fit into your family and belong. However, most parents of 2-year-olds are quite stressed, and chest breathing is a pattern of breathing that we adopt when we are stressed and overwhelmed. Unfortunately, it exacerbates the stress response and therefore the negative effects of stress on your body.

You can choose to switch back to full diaphragmatic, belly breathing all the time. It takes about 3 days of focus to change the habitual way you breathe to a more health enhancing pattern. You simply place your hands on your upper belly every time you think of it and breathe into your hands, so your belly expands and then as you release the breath your hands return toward your spine. If you do this regularly and consciously for a few days it becomes your usual unconscious way of breathing and then you can sit back and enjoy how much more energy you have, how calm you feel and a renewed sense of general well-being. You can teach your friends, family and children how to breathe in this way.

Regular practice of Makarasana, The Crocodile will also help to switch your usual breathing pattern to diaphragmatic or deep belly breathing. Don't force the breath, or overly expand the belly, your breathing should be relaxed, natural and easy.

When you breathe into your belly you are breathing with the diaphragm muscle. As you breathe in this muscle contracts and creates more space for the lungs to expand and as you breathe out it relaxes and gently pushes upward to help the lungs fully expel the air. See the diagram below.

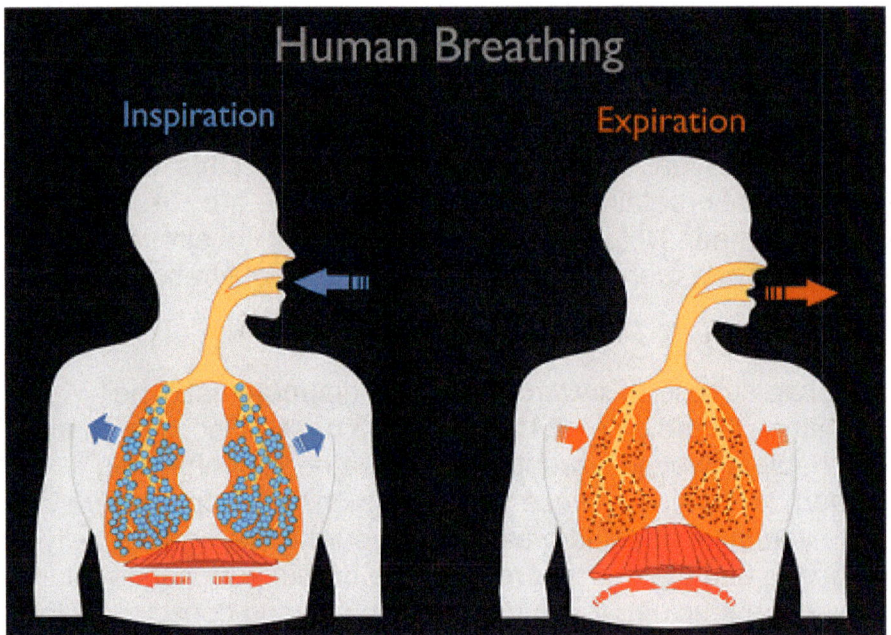

When we chest breathe the diaphragm moves upward with the inward breath restricting the lung capacity and moves downward with the out breathe so is unable to aid the full expulsion of air from the lungs. Diaphragmatic breathing is ideal for good health as you will discover, whereas chest breathing does not give you all these positive benefits and creates patterns in your body that are not conducive to optimal health.

Diaphragmatic or Deep Yogic Breathing takes your breath deeper and therefore slows the breath and the rate of breathing and gives your body more time to exchange oxygen for carbon dioxide in your lungs. So, each breath is more efficient.

The lower half of your lungs is where the tissue is most compacted and where most of the oxygen and carbon dioxide exchange occurs. By breathing deep into the lungs, you ensure more oxygen is absorbed and able to travel through your bloodstream to your heart to be pumped to every one of the trillions of cells in your body. It also relaxes tight chest muscles which further increases your lung capacity and subsequent oxygenation of all your cells.

This naturally improves your health, your vitality and especially your energy levels. It is estimated that we take between 17280 and 23040 breathes each day, so even a small increase in the efficiency of each breath equates to a big increase in your oxygen delivery and energy efficiency over the course of a day.

The Deep Yogic Breathing practiced in Makarasana strengthens the diaphragm muscle. When we chest breathe or have dysfunctional breathing patterns or suffer with conditions that compromise your breathing like COPD (Coronary obstructive pulmonary disorder) or Asthma the diaphragm is often weak, so strengthening this muscle can really help to improve the efficiency of your breathing.

In dysfunctional breathing patterns and Asthma your lungs lose their elasticity and don't contract fully with the out breath, so don't expel all the air. This leads to a build-up of air in the lungs, which means there is less space for the diaphragm to breathe in the air in the next breath, forcing your body to engage the neck, back and chest muscles to help get more air into the body. Strengthening the diaphragm and learning to relax and breathe deeply vastly improves these conditions.

The diaphragm attaches to the lumbar vertebrae in your lower back, to the tip of the breastbone and to the ribs, separating the chest cavity from the abdominal cavity. In Makarasana your body is forced to breathe deeply from the belly as the position immobilises the chest and forces you to use the diaphragm. Constrained by the floor and tightness across your chest and upper back the breath fills the lower back and sides of the waist. This will help to release any tension that has built up in the muscles in the lower ribs, back and waist area. It is not uncommon to have habitual tension in this part of your back, yet we become so used to it that we only notice when it is released or releasing.

With diaphragmatic breathing not only does your rate of breathing slow down, but it slows your heartbeat and can lower or stabilise your blood pressure. These are both very positive benefits to maximise the efficiency of your whole cardiovascular system and enhance your overall health.

Many people chronically mouth breath rather than nose breathing, even when their nose is not blocked. Again, this is a habit. Mouth breathing tends to dry the mucous membranes and gives less protection from the 20 billion particles that we are exposed to every day, many of which are potential pathogens. When we breathe through the nose it acts as a filter to capture bacteria, dust, and microbes, while warming and increasing the humidity of the air so that the breath flows easily. The increased resistance to the air stream helps to slow the exhalation rate down and optimise your oxygen uptake, increasing it by as much as 10-20%. This enhances your energy levels and health through the increased oxygenation of all your tissues.

'As you start to walk on the way

The way appears'

Rumi

Positive Effects on Stress and your Nervous System

Makarasana works positively to relax your nervous system and naturally promote relaxation, repair and rejuvenation.

Your nervous system is a communication network of nerves that runs throughout your body and enables your brain to keep your body functioning optimally and maintain a state of balance or homeostasis.

The Autonomic nervous system has two predominant states that set off a series of reactions and processes in the body depending on how we are responding to our environment. These are the sympathetic and the parasympathetic nervous systems, both of which are usually stimulated involuntarily by centres in our brain.

The Sympathetic nervous system is responsible for the fight or flight or in some cases freeze mechanism designed to protect and ensure your survival when you are threatened or perceive potential danger to your life.

This responds to your perception of danger, so it reacts not only to actual threatening or demanding situations in your external environment but also perceived threats and any associated thoughts about these situations in your internal or mind environment. This is how we can think or worry ourselves into a stress response that may or may not be happening. The tiger threatening your life may be in your mind rather than attacking you.

This attack may or may not be real, it may simply be something you are worried may occur or you may have exaggerated the threat as your mind spirals into projections of past experiences. The key thing to realise about stress is your body responds in the same way regardless of whether a tiger is ready to pounce or the tiger is something in your mind generating worrying thoughts about what might happen.

The sympathetic system is responsible for releasing the adrenaline and cortisol and other chemicals that are produced in response to stress which increase your heart rate and blood pressure, and divert the blood supply away from the digestive, growth and repair processes and toward the heart, lungs and big muscles ready for action. We feel 'wired to respond', in a heightened state, physically, emotionally and mentally. This state can become addictive when people live their lives in a constant state of stress and challenge.

This is fine as a short-term acute reaction and response to a threat, but harmful to your health if there is long term activation of the stress response and you are living in this chronic stressed, reactive survival state much of the time.

In this chronic state cortisol and other stress hormones are produced in high levels that disrupt almost all your body's processes. These can over time produce fatigue, irritability, headaches, intestinal problems like bloating, constipation and diarrhoea, weight gain, increased blood pressure, low libido, erectile dysfunction, menstrual and ovulation problems, difficulty recovering from exercise, poor sleep, impaired glucose/insulin metabolism, suppressed immune function and increase your risk of Anxiety and Depression.

Now let's look at the other state our nervous system can adopt. When the Parasympathetic nervous system is activated, you feel calm and chilled, and your body concentrates on processes involving growth and repair. This network controls everyday processes like food digestion, breathing rate, heart rate, blood pressure, body temperature and keeps your body in a state of homeostasis or balance and optimum health.

When you consciously breathe slowly and deeply you stimulate the Vagus nerve that <u>voluntarily</u> activates the parasympathetic nervous system so that your body can relax, heal and repair. This brings your heart rate, breathing rate and blood pressure down and promotes digestion, assimilation of nutrients, overall physiological repair processes and a healthy immune system.

We call this the Relaxation response. In addition, this response has been found to reduce muscle tension, fatigue, chronic pain, anxiety and improve memory and immune function.

Through regular voluntary activation of the Vagus nerve through deep relaxation you develop increased Vagal Tone, which means your body can relax faster and return quickly to a normal healthy state after you have experienced stress. You develop a resilience to stress. It takes more threat to elicit the stress response and grants you protection from the negative physical effects of stress in general. You experience stress as short term acute episodes rather than a long term, chronic, normal way of being.

Remember not all stress is negative, we often need a heightened state mentally, emotionally and physically to achieve our best performance or to push ourselves to grow or to find the courage to do what is needed. The key to our health resides in ensuring we do not become overly reactive to life's challenges or addicted to a highly charged state of being and have sufficient down time to relax, repair and recharge.

By spending time in Makarasana, you activate the parasympathetic nervous response and decrease the sympathetic nervous system response. Over time the sympathetic nervous system becomes less reactive, and the parasympathetic nervous system takes the driving seat becoming your default response to life. This shift improves your overall health and well-being by reducing the amount of stress you experience. People around you will notice, you are calmer, less reactive, more accepting and forgiving and start to take greater care of your health.

You will naturally feel more able to cope with and respond calmly to the challenges that life inevitably throws your way.

The relaxation response sends a positive signal to your body that you are 'safe' and this has been shown to promote higher states of functioning, improved healing and regeneration, and sustained feelings of fulfilment.

You move from Sympathetic Surviving
to Parasympathetic Thriving

Instead of being in a survival state when the sympathetic nervous system is dominant you switch to a state in which you thrive when the parasympathetic nervous system becomes your natural state.

This enhanced resilience to stress and better response to the challenges in your life is not just physical. You build emotional and mental resilience. This is something I have observed time and again in people that regularly practice yoga and especially Makarasana. I will talk more about this.

Deep Yogic or Belly breathing is an effective way to calm the rapid, shallow chest breathing associated with an anxiety or panic attack. By taking the breath deeper into your belly and slowing it down, this calms your mind and allows the parasympathetic system to bring your body back into a calm relaxed state. If you suffer with anxiety, with time and practice deep yogic breathing will enable you to calm your body if an anxiety attack has been triggered or avoid a full-blown attack when you first feel the warning signs. Dropping down into Makarasana if comfortable during or after the attack will help you to return to a calm, confident state easily and allow you to release the heightened emotions that naturally arise when you are in the grip of the overwhelming panic. Over time this will ease the frequency and severity of your attacks, as you develop an enhanced resilience to stress through increased parasympathetic vagal tone and a reduction in the sensitivity of your sympathetic nervous system. By spending time in Makarasana after the attack you can witness and release the fear patterns in your mind that are setting off the panic reaction. It provides a means to see and potentially heal the often-unconscious causes.

Digestive, Lymph and Immune System Health Benefits

Diaphragmatic breathing through its parasympathetic response optimises and maintains healthy digestive function. In a calm relaxed state, your body diverts your blood flow and energy to the gut to augment breakdown, and absorption of your food, ensuring you receive all the nutrients possible. The action of the diaphragm in breathing has a massaging effect on many of your internal organs and increases the blood flow to the intestinal tract helping to maintain good gut peristalsis, creating an ideal movement of substances through the tract and maximising absorption of nutrients and the removal of waste products. This can prevent acid reflux, bloating, intestinal spasms, constipation, and hiatus hernia and create a happy healthy digestive system.

Our digestive system is more complex than was previously thought and has a huge impact on whole-body health. A healthy gut contributes to a strong immune system, heart health, brain health, improved mood, healthy sleep, as well as effective digestion. There is a high correlation between digestive and gastro-intestinal issues and the imbalances in the brain neurotransmitters that are thought to be involved in Anxiety and Depression. This is a fascinating and quite new area of research into the significance of our gut health and especially the effect of the makeup of your unique gut bacterial population or gut micro biome. If you are interested, you can read more about this in any reputable up to date literature on this topic.

This massage effect of diaphragmatic breathing also helps to detoxify your body by stimulating the lymphatic movement in the whole abdominal cavity.

One of the major functions of the lymph system is to collect up excess fluid and return it to the bloodstream via a vessel in your chest, while flushing out toxins in your body in the process. Lymph contains amongst other things many immune white blood cells and these are concentrated in the lymph nodes that are a vital part of your immune system. The lymph doesn't have its own pump and so relies on muscle action to keep it flowing effectively. Deep yogic breathing helps to promote effective and healthy lymph flow and its detoxing actions by acting as a body pump returning the lymph back toward the chest and into the bloodstream.

Studies have shown that deep slow breathing helps both the lungs and the brain to optimise and maintain the blood ph. levels. Blood acidity is neutralised with the release of carbon dioxide from the lungs. Optimal oxygen exchange deep in your lungs facilitates this management of your body acidity. For ideal health your body cells function in an alkaline environment. When the acidity increases you are more susceptible to chronic disease that results from inflammation. Again, if you are interested, you can read more on this in any reputable up to date literature on this topic.

Positive Brain Wave States

Your brain waves can be measured by EEG recording equipment. Depending on what you are doing and your state of mind, your brain waves will oscillate at different frequencies.

When you are awake, alert, at ease and calm you are in an alpha brain wave state. In this state you can form a bridge between the conscious and the unconscious mind which is so important in healing emotional issues from your past. The alpha brain wave state is quite a creative state of mind allowing you to access solutions to problems quite beyond your normal everyday thinking processes.

As you begin to focus, listen, think and analyse, make decisions and process information about your environment you move into lower beta brain wave frequencies. If your thoughts become anxious, with increasing agitation you move into higher beta frequencies and experience the negative brain fog and inability to focus and remember that we associate with feeling 'stressed'. This is your brain going into nervous system overload.

As you relax in Makarasana you will naturally move from a beta brain wave state into the alpha state and if you are able to relax even deeper, you will move into an even slower theta brain wave state.

Theta brain waves are strong during any type of internal focus, during daydreaming, meditation or prayer. They are associated with the state between wakefulness and sleep and are only experienced briefly by most awake adults as they fall asleep each night. They are normal and predominant in children up to the age of 13 years and during lighter sleep in adults.

A theta brain wave state is highly desirable as in this state both your body and your mind experience enhanced rejuvenation, growth and healing. This is especially important if you have been ill, or experienced physical or mental 'burnout'. In the theta state you can create a bridge between the conscious and unconscious mind and open to ideas, solutions and understandings that come from a higher source, wisdom we call intuition (your inner tuition).

Relaxing deeply in Makarasana gives you the opportunity to drop down into this theta brain wave state and remain there for an extended time. This is one of the reasons I recommend you stay in Makarasana for 10 minutes and at least once a week use my Guided Relaxation to remain in this posture for 20 minutes to maximise your time in a theta brain wave state.

During periods when your life is quite stressful and you are suffering with symptoms of chronic stress, anxiety, depression or insomnia I would recommend you spend at least 10 minutes in Makarasana every day.

As you move into the state of mind associated with both alpha and theta brain waves you can access your unconscious mind, while increasing your ability to connect to and feel your emotions. It is in this state that you open to powerful mind-body healing and can become aware of and reprogram the conditioned responses, beliefs and values you find in your unconscious mind.

Your mind is like a computer; your brain is the hardware that downloads the programs you need for life and stores them on your hard drive. Your unconscious mind is this hard drive. We spend the first seven years of our life downloading these programs based on our experiences in our family and the world around us. Many of these programs serve us well as we navigate life but equally many are self-sabotaging, disempowering and contain limiting beliefs. As we mature and age life will present us with opportunities to witness these limiting beliefs. Our relationships with others are often the mirror that life holds up for us to see these unconscious programs; but only if you are willing to look. If you are caught up in your thoughts and not giving the present moment your full attention you will miss these golden opportunities. By simply 'seeing' them as the adult you are now, you are bringing them into your consciousness and then you can start to clear out that hard drive and re-program it with beliefs, attitudes and behaviours that are emotionally intelligent and serve you well in life.

We do this when we consciously use affirmations to reprogram our unconscious mind for example.

These relaxed states are the key to changing your habitual thought patterns and experiencing the positive benefits this inevitably brings in your life. So much of your behaviour, especially our reaction when we feel pressured or overwhelmed, stems from beliefs, attitudes, and values we hold in our unconscious mind. Going inward in Makarasana gives you the chance to see these patterns and their origins, let them go and consciously change them. This develops your self-awareness; your awareness of all aspects of you, hidden and unhidden.

The Theta brain wave state reduces stress and anxiety and boosts your immune system. It has been found to enhance your creativity and help advanced problem solving and learning ability. It seems to be the state in which we process emotional information and create memories. Theta brain wave activity has been measured when people report feeling an increased spiritual connection. This state has a very definite positive effect on our brain and nervous system health.

In teaching many yoga classes over the years I have observed that some people have trouble relaxing during the Deep Relaxation at the end of the class. They mention that their minds whirl and won't switch off and their body's twitch with restless energy and they just can't seem to let go and simply relax. I have been pleased to notice that within a few weeks of doing a 20 minute Deep Relaxation just once a week, this changes and they are able to relax deeply, remain in this state and learn to dive deep into the feeling of surrender and peace. They seem to fine tune their relaxation response, learning to relax quite naturally, like they did as a child. I often get reports that they experience the best sleep the night after class.

It is lovely to see the change in people when they learn to relax and surrender in this way. They return to sitting after the relaxation with a smile on their face, a sparkle in their eyes, calm and happy. I can see how much they enjoyed and benefitted from this simple practice. They look vibrant and younger as the tension has left their face.

When practiced at the end of a yoga class the Crocodile takes the benefits of the yoga postures held during the class deeper and allows the body to realign, harmonise and come back to balance following the energy shifts during the class.

Regular practice of Makarasana is excellent for restoring natural healthy sleep cycles especially if you struggle with insomnia or stress related sleep disturbances. When you have trouble getting to sleep at night or wake in the night and can't get back to sleep easily, practising Makarasana will help. You can lie on the floor in your bedroom if your mattress is not firm enough to do this posture in bed.

When you go to sleep relaxed both mentally and physically you improve the quality of your sleep, spending more time in the deeper restorative Delta brain wave state. The release of physical tension enables your body to relax and optimises the restorative and regenerative processes that are needed every night. Recent studies have found that sufficient sleep keeps you sharp, creative, attentive and able to process information quickly; whereas poor sleep can make you more likely to focus on negative information when making decisions and adversely affects your memory. During deep sleep your brain goes through a clearing, filing, restoring process that improves your memory function the next day. Interrupted or inadequate sleep is a major factor in the development of depression. Poor quality sleep has recently been linked with increased levels of the inflammatory processes that lead to many diseases in your body. You can see that getting adequate rest and relaxation as well as good quality sleep are essential to optimise your mental, emotional and physical well-being.

Creating a Meditative Mind

> 'When meditation is mastered,
>
> the mind is unwavering like
>
> the flame of a candle in a windless place'
>
> Bhagavad Gita

Through a gentle focus on your breath as you practice Makarasana you can take these health benefits even deeper and experience all the positive effects of the meditative state for your mind. There are numerous studies on the benefits of meditation and mindfulness for your mental, emotional and physical health but I would like to focus on the very tangible benefits you will experience in your mind.

You naturally weed the garden of your mind, negative thoughts are the weeds that wither and die through lack of attention, giving the positive thoughts, the flowers a chance to grow

Makarasana clears your mind, especially if you gently focus on the breath during the posture and allow the breath to take your mind inward to connect with a sense of stillness and peace. By continuing to focus on your breath you allow your mind to detach from the thoughts that run through your mind, and you can learn to simply observe them. In meditation we call this the state of the 'Silent Witness' or the' Silent Observer'.

As you continue this gentle focus on the breath, it changes your mind. You will experience fewer thoughts, with more space in between them. This brings a profound peace of mind and develops the discipline needed to allow you to drop down into deeper states of meditation and enjoy its power to positively change your mind. By returning to this focus on your breath whenever your mind is distracted you develop this capacity to step back and simply watch your thoughts pass through your mind. Every now and again you will get caught up in an enticing train of thought, but with practice you will recognise when your thoughts have wandered and learn to come back to a focus on the breath. I teach you to come back to this focus on your breath without judgement or criticism, but with an attitude of loving kindness.

We come to realise that we can't be our thoughts,

Because 'Who' is watching them?

Learning to detach from your usual thoughts gives you back the power to choose which thoughts you give your attention to and which you don't. If you think of the relentless thoughts that plague your mind every day, these are like powerful horses running wild. By detaching from your thoughts, you effectively take the reins and tame those galloping horses, bringing them back under control so that you can use their power to go where you want to go. In this way you take back control of your mind and can learn to use your mind as a powerful agent of positive change in your life.

The everyday thoughts that constantly run through your mind that Buddhist teachers call the chatter of the 'monkey mind', originate from your ego. Your ego is that part of your personality that wants to protect your idea of who you are and is reluctant to change even if that means you continue to suffer with thoughts that are not self-serving or self-affirming. As you learn to step back and simply witness these thoughts they lose their power. Instead, you connect with the Silent Witness, the Observer which is the wise aspect of you, often called your Higher Self or your Soul.

The space you create in your mind allows intuitive guidance, understandings and realisations to arise in your awareness. These come from a connection beyond your personality. As you learn to discriminate these gems of wisdom from your usual thoughts and trust them, you change. This is the secret and the power of meditation to change your mind and therefore change your life in amazing ways. I explore this in more detail in my online courses.

If you would like to explore a deeper understanding of the Power of Meditation, please visit my website teresa4yoga.co.uk/meditation or view the numerous meditation videos on my YouTube channel Teresa Keast.

If you feel drawn to explore a connection with the essence of your authentic Self, developing greater Self-Awareness I offer an online course entitled, Learn to Meditate through a Connection with Nature.
https://teresakeast.teachable.com/p/learn-to-meditate

You can experience greater peace of mind and all the joy and inner happiness that a practice of meditation naturally creates by learning to meditate in beautiful settings in nature.

An outer love of the peace in nature inspires an inner love of meditation and connection to a deep source of wisdom, clarity, calm and strength within you.

Includes comprehensive guidance and instruction from an experienced meditation teacher, videos in nature and audio mp3's to download and keep.

Subtle Energy, Chakra and Emotional Benefits

Makarasana has a beneficial effect on your subtle energy flow.

This is not the same as metabolic energy that we derive from the food we eat that powers our physical body. Subtle energy is experienced as our life force energy or our vitality. We assume in our culture that our vitality levels decline with age. However, many people who practice Yoga and other energy disciplines like Tai Chi or Qi gong that maintain the flow of subtle energy find this is not necessarily so.

We have an energy field that surrounds and interpenetrates our physical body. This field can be sensed, measured and photographed and constitutes a subtle energy or life force energy that infuses our physical body with vitality and gives it life. This energy is often referred to as Prana, Chi or Ki and people vary greatly in the vibration of their subtle energy depending on their state of being in any given moment and their emotional, mental, and spiritual health.

We know that this energy body or aura surrounds all living things and is where we experience the interplay and connection energetically with the energy of other living things in our environment. We are connected energetically to everything, from the smallest atom to stars and planets in the cosmos. All of life is interpenetrated by subtle energy in what many scientists now call the 'Unified field'. There is much written to support the idea that when we connect inwardly, we are connecting to this field and come into synchronisation with the energy of life, and this is where we find our potential to attract healing energies into our life that create positive change.

We sense this energy in a room where there has been a conflict, we sense when someone is feeling down even though they say they are fine, or we know some people just leave us feeling drained after we have been in their presence. We read this energy in others all the time even if we don't realise this and we feel it when we connect with our pets, animals, and the natural world.

We are naturally intuitive

when it comes to sensing energy

Our subtle energy travels in channels called meridian energy lines throughout the body recognised in Chinese and Ayurvedic medicine. Subtle energy or Prana enters the body through the chakra energy centres we have come to understand through Eastern Yoga Philosophy.

As Western Science explores the frontier between the physical and the subtle energy, this energy is being increasingly recognised for its importance in the health of our physical body. There are now many healing modalities that work to heal the physical body through clearing, rebalancing and rejuvenating the human energy field or energy pathways.

If you would like to explore an understanding of the Chakras and our Subtle Energy in depth, please view the following playlists on my YouTube channel. Note some of these talks are followed by a Group meditation for World Peace and Harmony.

Teresa Talks on Insights into the Chakras

Teresa Talks on Understanding Subtle Energy and Energy Dynamics

An understanding of your chakras is a vast subject. I will give you a brief overview or taste of this amazing wisdom as it relates to Makarasana.

Chakras are vortices or centres that allow subtle energy into your body in direct proportion to your spiritual development. Each chakra has associated with it, an element, colour, and relates to specific areas of your emotional, mental, and spiritual growth. Energy moves between the seven major chakra centres associated with the spine along invisible energy pathways we call nadis and this flow is enhanced when we practice certain yogic breathing, including the deep yogic breathing in Makarasana. This has a positive effect in keeping this energy and our vitality and subsequent growth and development moving and flowing.

In ancient wisdom teachings and many complementary and eastern health paradigms like Chinese Medicine, Ayurvedic Medicine, Homeopathy, Acupuncture, Naturopathy, Herbalism, Flower remedies, Reiki, Sound healing and other energy medicine modalities, dis-ease is created in the body when subtle energy doesn't flow. The disruption of the subtle energy in your body eventually manifests as physical symptoms that we diagnose and treat using our Western Medical approach. There is inherent in these health paradigms a belief that many dis-ease states originally had an emotional or mental causal element that blocked the flow of subtle energy resulting in the presentation of a condition in the physical body. I will explore this in more detail and how Makarasana helps to keep this subtle energy flowing and its positive effects on several key chakras.

Makarasana opens the Root Chakra, Muladhara, which is found at the base of your spine and associated with the earth element. It grounds or connects your energy to that of the Earth, our planetary home.

When you feel grounded you feel in touch with what is important. You feel connected to nature, and its seasons and cycles. This connection enhances your physical health, your immune system and naturally reduces any emotional or mental stress. It brings a sense of security and safety and a feeling like you fundamentally 'belong'. It is associated with high self-esteem and self-mastery.

Science now recognises that when you spend time in nature you come into tune with the Schuman resonance (7.83 Hz), which is the vibrational frequency of the Earth, or the heartbeat rhythm of our planet. This resonance creates many positive health benefits including the induction of a theta brain wave relaxed state.

Being grounded is something we find attractive energetically in others as we sense they are in touch with what is important and are confident in themselves. As you ground your energy through your base chakra, you will develop a belief and trust that your basic needs for survival will be met, and this often manifests in a capacity to attract energy in the form of money and other forms of abundance into your life. It certainly develops a fundamental trust that life supports you.

Blockages or overstimulation of Muladhara often present as low self-esteem, needy, self-destructive, overly materialistic, fearful, bullying or physically foolhardy behaviour. Physical conditions like osteoarthritis, and poor immune response, mental spaciness and a lack of concentration or difficulty achieving goals are attributed to imbalances in this chakra.

But Makarasana does more than simply open your base chakra, and ground your energy, it also enhances the flow of energy through and communication between the seven major chakras associated with your spine. This keeps your subtle energy moving and enhances your vitality and overall health and well-being not just physically, but emotionally, mentally, and spiritually.

Makarasana also works strongly to stimulate especially your sacral chakra, Svadhisthana and your solar plexus, Manipura chakra and can transmute or shift negative energies that are blocked in these centres to either the throat or the heart chakras. Before I describe this process of emotional release and resolution let us explore these energy centres in a bit more detail.

Svadhisthana is found around the navel and is your centre of creativity and relationship with others. It is strongly activated in the Crocodile posture.

It is associated with your creative expression and the creation of new life, the unconscious, your emotions and especially any unconscious desires, including sexual desires. This centre represents your sexual power and its expression through sensuality. It is where we first experience duality in all aspects of life, our gender, and the expression of masculinity and femininity within our own nature.

The Hindu symbol is a six petalled lotus containing a white circle, (symbolising the element of water), a light blue crescent moon (represents change and growth) within which is a 'Makara' (a crocodile like creature). The same Makara or namesake of Makarasana.

Makarasana has the capacity to help you to navigate and heal aspects of yourself that relate to the sacral chakra especially in your most intimate and important relationships.

It brings up and helps you to resolve any issues to do with your sexuality, your intimate connections in relationships, and any physical problems with the bladder, prostate, sexual organs or lower back.

Water is supposed to flow and has great power when it does, but it causes problems when it is blocked. This chakra is about learning to flow with life and follow your aspirations, intuition, and passions allowing who you are in truth to flow out into the world in your own unique expression.

Water symbolises the emotions. The flow of emotion cleanses and heals our heart chakra. You can see the parallels here as Makarasana sets you free to express your emotions and learn to ride the waves of strong emotions without being swamped by them. Emotional expression is often blocked by fear. Fear you will not be heard, that your expression is inappropriate or will be rejected or judged. We suppress our true feelings especially when we struggle to find the right words or their intensity scares us, believing this is the best way to avoid embarrassment, conflict and feeling vulnerable.

Fear will close your heart chakra and the suppression of the flow of emotional energy causes blockages in your subtle energy pathways. As these blockages impede the flow of life force energy in your body; in time they will manifest as physical health symptoms. When emotional energy is not released, it doesn't just disappear, it must go somewhere. It gets stored in your subtle energy and eventually in your tissues. You may have heard the saying 'the issues are in the tissues'.

Through the connection of the heart with the mind in Makarasana, you can express emotional energy that was blocked in a safe way as you maintain a healthy perspective through a mind that is observing this process. This is the key to the magic. As you express the emotions you are connected to the strength, calm and courageous aspect of your true Self and all the wisdom that comes through your mind that reveals the truths about the situation that set off your emotional reaction. This provides the opportunity to heal the root cause of this reaction and open your heart chakra again. So instead of being immersed in fear avoiding the pain of expressing your hurt, you open to being healed through love. You return to connection with your truth which is a return to love.

I think of the mind in this instance as the surfboard that enables us to ride the waves of our emotions, we are the surfer who is up above, observing and experiencing that ride. Makarasana empowers the surfer.

Blocked subtle energy in both the base chakra and the sacral chakra can be a contributing cause of many lower back problems. It is no coincidence that we often suffer lower back issues after losing our job, a loved one, or experiencing major challenges within our most sacred intimate relationships. All these life experiences challenge our feelings of security, safety and trust in others and in life itself.

Unbalanced energies in Svadhisthana can be associated with being emotionally unbalanced, manipulative, overly sensitive, feeling guilty or critical of yourself and others. It can manifest in sexual addiction, or problems with healthy sexual expression.

When the creative energies flow and Svadhisthana is in balance we are creative, expressive, passionate, attuned to our own feelings and naturally trusting. We express our authentic self in all aspects of our life and are 'happy in our own skin'.

A regular practice of the Crocodile posture keeps your sacral chakra in balance which improves the flow of creative energy in your body including the sexual energy and its healthy expression.

It is a natural development for the creative energies of the sacral chakra to rise to the throat chakra Vishuddha, allowing us to express our creativity through truthful communication and the expression of ideas. It is my belief that this movement of energy is a natural process that occurs for women during the menopause and that many menopausal symptoms are a result of the inhibition of this energy flow. Makarasana will help this flow.

Manipura, the solar plexus chakra is your centre of passion, fire and will energy associated with the fire element, self-empowerment and transformation.

Physically it is associated with your digestive organs and imbalances often present as stomach, gall bladder, liver, or other digestive problems, weight gain especially around your torso or diabetes.

Emotionally imbalances can present as insecurity and a fear of being alone or an over concern with what others think of you. But primarily this chakra is associated with anger and especially unresolved or unexpressed feelings of anger, irritation, resentment, and frustration. When Manipura is out of balance we can come across as angry, controlling or needing to be in control, judgemental and superior. There can be a propensity to seek solace in addictive behaviours, eating, drinking, taking drugs, excessive shopping or becoming a 'workaholic'. These addictive life habits can be a way of avoiding facing these strong feelings.

When your Manipura chakra is in balance you exhibit a natural respect for yourself and others, spontaneity, and healthy personal power.

One of the most powerful benefits of Makarasana is its capacity to shift this build-up of unresolved issues around anger, personal power and the right use of your will energy and move it up into your heart chakra Anahata to be resolved.

When this occurs you may experience an actual physical release of energy which may bring tears, and a feeling that a heavy burden has been lifted and an easing of tension around the solar plexus area of your body.

If you can remain in Makarasana through this process of emotional cleansing, healing and release, the energy that was blocked starts to flow up into the higher chakras and because your forehead is touching your hands and stimulating the Ajna or third eye chakra, this enables you to intuitively see or understand the situation from a different perspective. It literally opens another eye, your third eye or inner eye so you can see the whole drama in a new light.

Often you will experience a dawning or a sudden realisation of your part in a conflict you had held anger or a grudge over for years. You may see the others person's point of view or see that although they made a mistake or didn't treat you well, they were doing their best and dealing with challenges you could not appreciate at the time.

If you are open to this flow of truthful insight it will enable you to come to a place of acceptance of past grievances and to gain understanding into what was really playing out at the time. You can see past the drama to the truth of the situation, and it can be quite revealing and even humbling.

It connects us to the 'essence' of our humanity

and gives us the power to extend this to others

You ultimately come through acceptance to forgiveness. In forgiveness you don't have to condone another's or your own behaviour, but you can open your heart and forgive them anyway and eventually forgive yourself for any part you played or for simply holding the grievance for so long.

Through this process of coming to acceptance and forgiveness and opening to the healing energy of your heart centre you can set yourself free of this issue forever. You don't have to involve the other person at all; it doesn't require difficult conversations or contact with them. This is all about your healing and simply taking responsibility for your own mental, emotional, and physical health. It naturally promotes your own spiritual growth and development as a person. As you come to realise your connection with all living things you also realise that forgiveness is ultimately about forgiving yourself. When you hold onto the anger, resentment, or other negative emotions you are only harming yourself. By choosing to release these, you are healing yourself.

The wonderful thing is that because we are all connected on some level you are helping the other person or people involved to heal as well. I think of it like a game of 'tug of war', while you hold the grievance you experience all the strain of years of pulling on the conflict, insisting that the way you see things is the whole truth. When you simply let go of the rope the tension evaporates and you are free, this opens you up to greater truths and realisations. You may need to pick yourself up off the ground as you process this new information, but you can walk away with your head held high and your heart healed. As you let the rope go the other party involved in the conflict are also set free; however, what they do with that is up to them.

I have witnessed what I would call miraculous healing when people let go difficult traumas and issues, they have carried for years through spending time in Makarasana and being open to embracing this process and surrendering to the magic of this posture to return them to emotional balance and well-being. Sometimes you will let go issues and not even be aware of what they were, but just that you have let something negative and uncomfortable go as you feel a lifting of the burden, your energy flow and your sense of well-being return.

This is the power of this posture to heal major trauma and to restore the natural joy and fulfilment, gratitude, and openness we find in people who have faced major issues and had the courage to open their heart and move forward.

The solar plexus is the seat of the Warrior in Yoga, and it takes a courageous heart to face these issues and lift the energy from the Manipura chakra up into Anahata, the heart chakra where it is transmuted. You are asked to step into your vulnerability when you open your heart and this can feel uncomfortable at first, until you come to know that your vulnerability is your greatest strength as a human being.

But you must be prepared to let go and be open to the light of understanding and accept healing and a new perspective.

You take responsibility for our own emotional, mental, physical and spiritual healing

You can choose to hold onto your anger and your version or story of what happened and the superior feelings of being right and knowing you were 'wronged'. This is always a choice. But it will block your natural subtle energy flow and life will keep bringing up drama's that encourage you to address this issue. Or you can embrace this natural process of change and transformation. Makarasana presents you with a choice, to end the suffering and open to joy and really live a heartfelt life.

A good example is to use Makarasana to improve depression. From a Yoga understanding of the relationship between the mind and the body, depression is a major blockage in the subtle energy flow that is ultimately caused by blocked anger, resentment or frustration. These emotions or energies were not expressed or not able to be expressed at the time and the negative energy that was suppressed gets stuck and causes a blockage in the solar plexus chakra and this area of the body. This impedes the flow of life force energy and damps down your will or fire energy, creating overwhelming fatigue and a crippling inability to pick yourself up emotionally and mentally. You lose your will power and your passion for life. Makarasana creates a gentle pressure on the solar plexus area that can help to release this blocked energy and the original emotions that caused it, over time, allowing the subtle energy to flow again, restoring vitality, passion, and the power of your will.

Igniting your will creates the desire and impetus for change while the enhanced vitality provides the energy needed to act. The connection established to the unconscious mind through retreating inward for answers, allows you to see the situation that caused the anger in a new light. Opening to an understanding of your part in the drama and acceptance of the part others played. This acceptance can lead to forgiveness and healing as the blocked energies lift from the solar plexus centre to the heart centre.

Physically gut and blood sugar problems resolve, and your energy levels return, a bonus is often the excess weight carried around your middle starts to shift.

Heart Coherence

The position you adopt in Makarasana with your forehead on your hands or forearms with your chest open and elbows naturally bent connects the head and the heart. Whenever I have a decision to make in which my mind tells me one thing, but my heart is telling me another I spend time in Makarasana until the two come together and the right and true decision becomes apparent. It is often something I feel to be right, rather than I think is right.

Your heart is intelligent, recently scientists at the Heartmath Institute in America have found it has its own neural network and over 40 000 neural cells called neurites. Their studies have shown that you receive information through your heart even before your brain has registered what is going on in your environment and it has its own capacity to learn and remember.

The heart has its own electromagnetic field or energy field that communicates with every cell in your body, and the frequency of these energy waves depends on how you are feeling emotionally. Heartmath studies have found that habitual positive emotions can switch on health enhancing DNA in your cells and negative states of emotion can have the opposite effect.

When you lie in Makarasana and relax deeply and bring your awareness to your heart centre in the centre of your chest, you can tune into this intelligence. By spending four minutes breathing deeply with a feeling of gratitude or care or compassion in your heart you come into what the Heartmath Institute calls 'Heart Coherence'. In this state you bring your heart and mind intelligence into an integrated, synergistic, coherent connection, enabling them to work powerfully together.

You can access higher states of consciousness and memories, profound understanding, and insights that you could not have worked out by simply using the analytical, logical function of your mind alone.

Through this heart-mind connection you can consciously gain access to your unconscious mind allowing the opportunity to view and release any deeply held beliefs, conditionings, attitudes and values that no longer serve you.

So when you are at a crossroads in life, you could weigh up the pros and cons of a decision and this is of value, or you could tune in intuitively in this way, gain much insight and the perfect solution will be there for you, as if by magic, loud and clear and beautiful in its simplicity, its completeness. You will know it by an inexplicable sense that it is right and good and true. This is something you must experience to truly appreciate.

This capacity of Makarasana to naturally heal your emotional upsets and bring you back to balance is especially beneficial to those who are experiencing difficulties with expressing emotions. I have seen it calm teenagers quickly and bring them peace and understanding and had a mother of a highly functioning autistic boy come up to me after a children's yoga class begging me to show her what the Crocodile was as her son found so much benefit and was so calm and happy after being in this wonderful posture.

Simply Being

When we come into the present moment, mindful and aware, we are simply being. This connects us to life in this moment, to experiencing all the beauty moment by moment and powerfully restores our balance and equilibrium. When we are mindful and present in this moment in time, we feel happy and content.

By resting in the Crocodile we are simply 'Being'

This restores balance to a life of busy 'Doing'

Try looking around you and simply being present to all that is going on in this moment. Listen to the sounds, notice how your body feels, allow the tastes and smells of this moment to enter your awareness. Give what is, your full attention. Whenever your mind starts to analyse, criticise or start a story about this moment, simply let this go and return to the experience of the moment. Notice how beautiful and alive and peaceful the world is when you give it your full awareness. In this moment everything is always fine. In this present moment you can change, in fact this is the only time and opportunity you have to change. You are not preoccupied with the past and all your reactions and regrets, with their associated fears and doubts and you are not projecting these into the future as worries and anxieties.

You are simply responding to life as it is.

Practising mindfulness develops your self-awareness and enhances your self-honesty and reflection and is essential to truly connecting with your Self as well as authentically connecting with others. When you are not caught up in your thoughts you bring your essence, your Soul, your Presence into the present moment and this creates an experience of truth, beauty and goodness.

Yin and Yang Balance

In Makarasana there is another subtle level of restoration of balance or equilibrium that naturally occurs. It allows the yin, feminine, reflective energy of being to balance with the yang, masculine, expressive energy of doing.

This balance is essential to good health from a Taoist point of view and in my own experience I find by spending time in the Crocodile I nourish my inner feminine and this restores my energy so that I am more creative and effective when I go out into the world and express my masculine side in doing what I need to do.

Relating to my previous discussion of being and doing, 'to be' is feminine and 'to do' is masculine, and when these are in balance health and harmony prevail.

We all have feminine and masculine energies and the balance between them is vital if you want to be able to give and make a difference in your world and for those you care about and to receive love and nourishment from the world and those who care about you.

This is enhanced by the opening of the chest and therefore the opening of the heart chakra in this posture. When we are open-hearted, we develop trust, courage and this restores our capacity to both give and receive love.

Without sufficient time to restore and balance in this way my life would easily become one of constant giving and doing and, in my experience, this quickly leads to exhaustion. This is a lesson I have had to learn the hard way; by over doing and giving to others my body eventually forced me to recharge and receive through illness and chronic fatigue. A breakdown in this way is often a breakthrough to realising how our life is out of balance, and it forces us to look at how we are living and whether there is a balance between expressing our feminine and masculine and to make the changes needed to restore this balance and our health. This has a powerful effect on balancing our hormones for both men and women and particularly so at times in your life when your hormonal system is going through major changes, like puberty or the menopause.

As we restore the balance within our self, often this restoration brings healing to our most intimate relations with others.

By spending time simply being, reflecting and relaxing in

Makarasana

I find I am more efficient when I return to do

what I need to in the world

I mentioned earlier that the Svadhisthana chakra symbol contained the makara within a blue crescent moon. This posture has an affinity to the divine feminine quality of the lunar energy that is a deeply reflective, intuitive, nurturing, and nourishing energy. The moon often represents that which is hidden, or unconscious to our present awareness. Esoterically the full moon is a time that has the potential to reveal and ultimately heal that which is hidden. In the energy of the new moon, we implement the desired changes as a result. So, by spending an extended time in Makarasana we allow these unconscious aspects of our nature to arise into our conscious awareness.

The moon has the power to move the water in the oceans on our planet and likewise it has the power to affect the flow of emotions within us. Our planet is 70% water and so is our body so it makes sense that we would be affected by the lunar cycles. Often people feel quite emotional and may not sleep well, around the time of the full moon and so it is particularly important to employ the magic of Makarasana at this time.

Self-Empowerment and a Life of Meaning and Purpose

'The meaning of life is to give life a meaning'

Victor Frankl

When we take responsibility for our physical, emotional, mental and spiritual health we are naturally stepping away from handing over the responsibility for our happiness and our health to others. We are effectively choosing to walk a path that involves self-autonomy and owning our sovereignty as spiritual beings having a human experience. By taking the step to relax into a posture that will help you to surrender that which you are not you are opening to realising that which you are. Your magnificence…

Through having the courage to begin to delve into that which still needs redeeming in your unconscious psyche you are embarking on a journey that while tough at times is truly rewarding as it enables a life of true meaning. We come to understand the idea that rather than looking for our path in life we realise that we are the path, and our life is an expression of who we are. There is a feeling of truly 'living' your life, a sense of aliveness that comes with the vitality of emerging into the light of your true being. This sense of quiet inner confidence and self-assurance is precious beyond measure. You ignite the warrior within and come to realise that challenges in your life are simply there to enable you to develop and grow stronger or reveal capacities and capabilities you didn't realise you had within you.

This sense of self-empowerment cannot be taken from you. It comes from within and is not dependent on anything external to you or anyone else in your life. The true beauty of this sense of inner empowerment is that by radiating your light you enable others to find their light. Your energy radiates out from your true self and unconsciously helps those around you to heal, to find purpose and meaning simply by being in your presence. You become a shining beacon to those you care most about.

All of this from trusting an amazingly simple yoga posture and letting it become your friend and guide whenever life gets tough or you need a break or to relax.

I hope and trust that this deep dive into the wisdom and understanding of this simple, humble, but immensely powerful posture Makarasana, the Crocodile encourages you to make it a part of your life.

It is my deepest hope that you will experience all the benefits I have outlined in this book and more. That you will use it regularly to relax and call upon its power when you feel in crisis and in need of understanding, love and support from your Highest Self.

Please teach it to your children, your family and anyone you know who might benefit from its transformative magic. This way together we can spread this magic and make a difference to the lives of many.

In essence Makarasana relaxes you physically, brings you back to peace emotionally, understanding mentally, connects you with your truth spiritually and restores balance and harmony on all levels of your being.

In choosing Makarasana you choose to thrive,

rather than simply survive.

So let the Magic of Makarasana transform your life today

Namaste Teresa

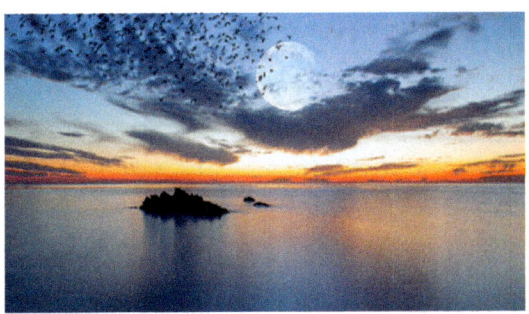

Connect with Teresa

If you enjoyed the insights and experience of this book and would like to take your exploration further, you could connect with my work in the following ways:

Explore my YouTube channel, or connect on linkedin, or substack, search 'Teresa Keast'

Connect with me on facebook and Instagram, search 'Teresa4Yoga'

Visit my website 'teresa4yoga.co.uk' for a wealth of information on yoga, meditation, yoga dance, spiritual development, healthy eating, energy therapies, corporate courses, online courses or one to one sessions.

Thank you for taking the time to read this book and embark on this journey with me.

If you enjoyed it, please take a moment to leave me a review at your favourite retailer.

About the Author

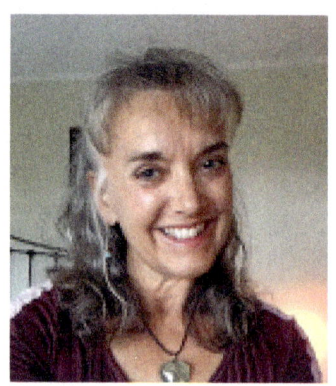

I am passionate about helping you transform your life through yoga, meditation, and a deeper spiritual understanding of who you are. This naturally cultivates a connection with an intuitive wisdom that guides, supports and enables the manifestation of your dreams.

With 30 years working in stress management, 20 years teaching yoga and meditation, self/spiritual development workshops and retreats, 35+ years meditating myself and studying ancient wisdom teachings and the science behind them, degrees in Physical Education and Nutrition and currently studying a Psychology degree I bring a depth of knowledge and experience.

I would love to help you enjoy more peace, confidence, health, vitality, fulfilment and happiness in your life, connecting with the Truth of who you are so that you can express **All That You Are**.

Knowledge becomes wisdom when it is practically applied, and I believe that understanding leads to positive change especially when combined with the very practical life changing techniques I love to teach.

I am a single mother of four beautiful now grown-up children, originally from New Zealand and would describe myself as open, friendly and down to earth with a love of the outdoors that is only rivalled by a passion to understand the deeper aspects of life, my love of yoga, meditation and teaching.

Through years of writing articles, blogs, giving talks, workshops and retreats this is my first foray into writing a book. It has been an exciting, sometimes frustrating but very worthwhile experience that I plan to repeat.

If it makes a difference, then I am very happy.

Namaste Teresa

***

Printed in Dunstable, United Kingdom